THE POISON DIET

INFORM YOURSELF BEFORE IT'S TOO LATE

A.L HARLOW

I0408176

INTRODUCTION

This book was written to help bring attention to the dangers of processed foods. Many people are unaware of the harmful chemicals they consume every day.

The FDA is not looking out for us, and manufacturers are not required to label dangerous additives in the foods they produce, no matter how bad they are.

With the knowledge you will gain from this book you will know what you are consuming and will be able to make intelligent choices regarding what you put in your mouth.

You and your family will live longer and stay healthier by not eating processed foods. Chemicals, like Glyphosate from Monsanto can be found in food, (even before processing) can give you cancer and other diseases.

Table Of Contents

WHAT ARE PROCESSED FOODS?

Food processing is the magical transformation of various ingredients by both physical and chemical methods into food, or the transformation of food into other forms.

Any processing of food will, in all likelihood, affect the food's nutritional value. How many nutrients are lost depends on both the food and processing method used. Consider the fact that heat destroys vitamin C. As a result canned fruits will give you less vitamin C than fresh fruits.

Food additives represent an additional concern for safety. The risks additives pose to one's health varies greatly from one individual to another. A prime example, is sugar, it endangers diabetics. Another is salt, it affects people with high blood pressure.

Not only microwave and other ready meals are processed foods. The phrase processed food, is in reference to any food that has been changed from its natural form in any way.

You may be consuming much more processed food than you are aware of.

Processed foods aren't by default unhealthy, but any food that has been processed might contain added salt, artificial flavoring, chemical preservatives, sugar and fat.

The major benefit of preparing food from scratch is that you know exactly what is going into it. However, even home cooked food often includes processed ingredients.

What is considered processed food?

You can be sure that most food bought in a shop has been processed in some form.

Here are some common processed foods.

Breakfast cereals
Cheese
Canned vegetables
Bread
Savory snacks including crisps
Meat products like bacon
Microwave meals or ready meals
Drinks, like milk or soft drinks

The techniques used in Food processing include canning, freezing, baking, pasteurizing and drying products.

When fruit and veg are frozen most of the vitamins are preserved, while tinned produce, without added sugar and salt, are convenient to store, cook and good to eat year round producing less waste and at a lower cost than fresh foods."

So what makes some foods less healthy when they are processed?

Additives like fat, salt and sugar are often added to processed foods to make them taste better and to extend shelf life.

This often leads to people consuming more than the safe amounts for these additives. This is because people may not know how much has been added to the food they are eating. These foods are frequently higher in calories because of the large amounts of added sugar or fat.

Furthermore, regularly eating more than 90g a day of red and processed meat has been linked to a greater risk of bowel cancer. Other studies have also indicated that eating large amounts of processed meat may be linked to an elevated risk of heart disease.

What is processed meat?

The term, "processed meat", means meat that has been preserved by curing, salting, smoking, or adding preservatives. Processed meats include bacon, sausages, ham, pâtés and salami.

The Department of Health recommends that you not more than 70g of red and processed meat a day. This equals a little over two slices of roast lamb, beef or pork or two or three rashers of bacon, with each being about equal in size to a half a slice of bread.

It's vitally important to remember that "processed" applies to a very broad range of food stuffs, many of which are okay to be eaten as part of a balanced diet.

How can I limit processed foods in my diet?

By reading the nutrition labels you will be able to make informed choices between processed products thereby keeping a close watch on the amount of processed foods that are high in fat, salt and added sugars that you are actually consuming.

Putting canned tomatoes in your shopping basket is a great way to improve your 5 a day. They can be stored longer and are less expensive than fresh tomatoes but first check the label to make sure they don't contain added salt or sugar.

Most of the pre-packaged foods have a nutrition label.

This nutrition label will include information on fat saturates, energy, carbs, protein, sugars and salt. The nutrition label may also give you information on nutrients such as fiber. Nutrition information is always based on a 100 gram serving and occasionally per portion.

How do I determine if a processed food is high in saturated fat, sugar or salt?

There are guidelines to tell you. These are:

Total fat
High = more than 17.5 grams per 100 grams
Low = 3 grams per 100 grams

Saturated fat
High = more than 5 grams per 100 grams
Low = 3 grams or less per 100 grams

Sugars
High = more than 22.5 grams per 100 grams
Low = 5 grams or less per 100 grams

Salt
High = more than 1.5 grams (or 0.6g sodium)per 100g
Low = 0.3 Grams (or 0.1g sodium) or less per 100g

If you are trying to reduce your intake of saturated fat, limit the amount of foods that contain more than 5 grams per 100g.

Some nutrition labels use color-coding that often show a mixture of red, amber and green. When you're trying to make a choice between similar products, to make a healthier choice, go for more greens and ambers, and fewer reds,.

Nevertheless, even the "healthier" ready meals will probably be higher in fat and other additives than what you would make at home.

THE 2 MILLION YEAR HISTORY OF PROCESSED FOODS

We're told it is the sinister force behind the epidemic of obesity, the demise of family farms and Tang. But in truth, humans have been creating processed foods since they learned to cook, freeze, ferment, preserve, extract and dry foods. Processed foods have driven the development of humans as a species, the growth of kingdoms and our exploration of our solar system. Here are the high-points.

Roasted Meat

Almost 2 million years ago we learned to enjoy roasted meat.

Fire-cooked food is much easier to digest and more nourishing than uncooked meat. Some anthropologists have put forth the argument that cooking was "the" crucial step that permitted humans to develop the big brains which is a characteristic of us Homosapiens.

Bread

Crop growing began somewhere around 12,000 years ago, but bread baking by early Europeans began many thousands of years before that then. In 2010 scientists found evidence of starch grains on rudimentary mortars and pestles at locations in Russia, Italy, the Czech Republic and Russia. These starches derived from the roots of ferns and cattails. Early humans pounded these into flour, mixed in water and baked a rudimentary form of bread.

Bread was an excellent dietary supplement because it was portable, nutrient-rich and did not spoil quickly. However, nutritionally speaking It was a step backward. Studies have shown that the Neolithic hunter-gatherers consumed a more wide-ranging and wholesome diet than Neolithic farmers. From the position of energy use, hunter-gatherers were far and away more organized. It would take a farmer ten hours to grow food containing the same amount of calories that only six hours of scavenging could provide.

So, a logical question; why bother with bread at all? Anthropologists have debated the question of why farming became dominant, but one thing is definite; bread and agriculture were inter-reliant. As social orders began to be dependent on bread as a key foodstuff, they were also forced to put more effort into agriculture.

Beer

The birth of beer is difficult to pin down. The oldest tangible indication came from pottery in Iran that date back to 5500 years ago, but archaeologists suggest that the first beer may have been brewed as long as 9000 years ago as a by-product of making bread. Early civilizations were quick to embrace the accidental discovery; it is presumed that the early

Sumerians might have diverted up to 40 percent of all grain produced into beer production.

Tortillas

Though there are no written records from before the date of the arrival in the Americas of Spanish explorers, early archaeological indications of maize farming dates back to about 8,700 years ago. Early Americans soaked kernels in a solution of lime to create masa, releasing beneficial nutrients during the process.

Wine

The earliest evidence of wine fermentation from about 7400 years ago has been found in the Zagros Mountains of Iran. Maritime Phoenicians spread the knowledge westward from Lebanon to Egypt and the Mediterranean.

Cheese

Place milk in a ruminant's stomach then agitate. It is thought by scholars that this is probably close to how cheese was invented. The earliest indications for cheese making were found in 7,000-year-old archaeological sites in Poland. Milk fat remnants were found in holed ceramic containers that are presumed to have served as basic strainers. It is entirely possible that with the domestication of sheep and goats as early as 10,000 years ago and of cattle 1,000 years later, it is possible that cheese production had been happening for longer.

Like other early foodstuffs, cheese was probably a product of necessity. Butter, yogurt and cheese, yogurt could be kept for a longer time than milk. Lactose was not digestible by Neolithic humans. The gene required for this adaptation has only spread as recently as the past few thousand years. The Bacteria that is used to make cheese ferments the milk lactose into lactic acid, thereby enabling easier digestion of dairy products.

Olive Oil
Raw olives are inedible due to their bitterness. However, farmers in the eastern Mediterranean began fermenting olives in lye and pressing them for oil for about 6,500 years.

Palm Oil
Palm oil is made from palm berries. Palm berries keep well on a shelf and are even today a cheap staple of processed food. Palm oil has been found in ancient Egyptian tombs dating back to 5,000 years ago.

Pickles
The ancient Mesopotamians of about 4,400 years ago were the first to store vegetables in vinegar thereby preserving them for consumption when they were out of season.

Noodles
The earliest evidence of this widespread food comes from unspoiled millet-based noodles found in an earthenware bowl in China dating to about 4,000 years ago. The wheat variety used to make pasta,

arose in China about 2,000 years ago and spread from there.

Chocolate

About 3,900 years ago pre-Olmec people in the Americas ground cacao beans, mixed in with water and stirred the mixture creating a foamy drink. 3,400 years later Hernando Cortés introduced the beans to Spain, where, for the first time, sugar was added.

Bacon

The first to salt pork bellies were Chinese cooks about 3,500 years ago. There were two reasons for this, preservation and a way to enhance the flavor of the meat.

Jiang

Jiang, created some 3,000 years ago, was the predecessor of flavor enhancers like miso and soy sauce. According to an ancient Chinese text, mixing meat or fish with salt and liang qu then leaving the mixture to mature for 100 days is how Jiang was made. As with many fermented foods, discovering it was probably an accident, but Jiang's spreading across East Asia was not. In the first to seventh centuries the rise of Buddhism throughout Asia in all likelihood brought Jiang to Korea and Japan.

Sugar

Sanskrit texts from India show that 2,500 years ago, cooks processed sugarcane into large crystals by boiling and cooling sugarcane juice. Nearly a thousand years later they invented granulated sugar, launching the global sugar trade.

Mustard

Among the earliest mustard recipes was one collected in a Roman cookbook. The recipe which is 2,400 years old, described a mixture of ground mustard seed, caraway, lovage, pepper, roasted coriander seeds, celery, thyme, dill, onion, honey, oregano, fish sauce, oil and vinegar.

Kimchi

Originally, kimchi was developed 2,700 years ago. It was cabbage fermented with salt. When the Japanese invaded Korea in the 16th century they took with them red chilies that had been introduced to them by the Portuguese missionaries who had brought it to Japan, afterwards Koreans started incorporating fiery elements into the dish.

Sushi

Sushi started 2,700 years ago as a means of fish preservation in Southeast Asia. Salted fish was covered in boiled rice and left to ferment for months. The rotted rice was scraped off and thrown away and the soured fish consumed. Due to the waste, sushi was always a dish for the wealthy. The process is similar to today's practice of dry-aging beef. During the 19th-century the long fermentation was replaced by adding vinegar into the rice mixture.

Tofu

The origins of Tofu are mysterious. The first written

record appears in the stories of Chinese writer Tao Ku from 2,900 years ago. He wrote about a vice mayor who was so poor, he had no choice but to buy tofu. Tofu is a coagulated gel made from cooked soybeans rather than mutton.

Salt Cod

Even though dried cod had been a staple food for the Vikings since the ninth century, in the tenth century salt changed it from a local food to a global marvel. With salt cod could be easily dried and preserved even in humid, wet or warm environments like a fishing boat. Over the next few hundred years salt cod supported the long journeys exploring the New World.

Peanut Butter

The Aztecs made a paste of ground uncooked peanuts in the 15th century.

Coffee

Coffee is a Western favorite, but it began in the Arab world. The most believable claim to the birth of coffee originates from Yemeni Sufi monasteries in the 15th century.

Coffee was first given for narcolepsy, torpor, stomachaches and other maladies. But coffee was not only curative; Arabic writers also noted its influences on socializing. For 16th century European travelers and explorers, coffee was an additional oddity of the Orient.

Carbonated Water

The British natural philosopher, Joseph Priestly, who discovered oxygen, created carbonated water after placing a bowl of water above a brewery in Leeds, England.

Corn Flakes

John Harvey Kellogg and his younger brother, Will Keith Kellogg, developed corn flakes in 1894 to gratify the vegetarian diet promoted by Seventh-Day Adventists.

MSG

In 1886 Karl Ritthausen, a German agricultural chemist discovered glutamic acid, of which MSG is just one variation.

Spam

In 1926 Hormel spiced ham was the first product of what ultimately became Spam. Originally it was cured pork shoulder in a can. Competition soon came along with their versions. To distinguish his creation, Jay Hormel changed the recipe in 1937 by mincing the pork, adding some salt and spices, and encasing the meat in gelatin. To this day, Spam remains a popular product.

Chicken Nuggets

In the 1950s Robert C. Baker, a food scientist minced chicken parts and coated them with bread as a way to increase the sale of chickens in New York state.

High-Fructose Corn Syrup

In 1806 the search for sugar alternatives began when

Napoleon Bonaparte offered a reward to any person who could find a chemical replacement for sugar due to the British blockade of the French Caribbean plantations. 150 years later American scientists found a way to use enzymes to convert glucose in cornstarch to fructose. Then in 1967 a Japanese scientist created a cost-efficient process. Food companies were enamored with the low cost and the simplicity of dissolving liquid corn syrup into sodas.

Tang

Tang was created in 1959 after scientists at General Foods had toiled for years attempting to create an orange juice substitute in powder form. All of their potions had an unpleasant, bitter taste. They found success when they abandoned their determination to include all of orange juice's vitamins and minerals.

Plumpy Nut

Plumpy Nut entered the scene in 1996 as a nutritious, vitamin strengthened product made from peanuts, powdered milk, vegetable oil, and sugar. Plumpy Nut was intended to help severely undernourished children gain weight.

Lab-Grown Meat

Lab-grown meat made its debut in 2013. The first taste test of in vitro meat for the public is planned to feature a burger grown from cattle stem cells.

1910s to 2010

Let's take a journey back in time and look at how we became a society where high-fat, fast, processed food has become so popular.

1910

In the 1890s trans fats were invented and became part of the food supply in the 1910s.

These delights came into being in the 1910s.

Nathan's hot dogs
Aunt Jemima syrup
Hellmann's mayonnaise
Oreo cookies
Crisco
Marshmallow Fluff

1920

Women were growing weary in the 1920s. They were weary of preparing foods as they always had and ready-to-cook foods were becoming more obtainable. New methods of food processing were brought about as a result of WWI. These included canned and frozen foods. Promising to save time for housewives were processed food ads. Kitchen tools, gas stoves, electric refrigerators and other appliances began to appear in more and more homes, this allowed more types of food to be purchased and stored. The taste buds were opened to new flavors, introduced by immigrants.

These delights came into being in the 1920s.

Baby Ruth candy bar
Wonder Bread

Yoo-Hoo beverage
VanCamp's canned pork and beans
Reese's peanut butter cups
Welch's grape jelly
Popsicles
Wheaties
Kool-Aid
Peter Pan peanut butter
Velveeta cheese

1930

With the great depression looming In the 1930s, families had to survive on less, watch their pennies and make food go further by reducing protein and including more vegetables.

Colonel Sanders developed his secret formula for spicing fried chicken at Sanders Court and Café in Kentucky.

These delights came into being in the 1930s.

Snickers Bar
3 Musketeers
Spam
Kraft Macaroni & Cheese
Ritz Crackers

1940

The 1940s required rationing in order to feed the soldiers fighting in WWII soldiers. Following the war, more convenience foods were introduced; dehydrated juice, instant coffee and cake mixes. Adding more conveniences, Tupperware and aluminum foil were presented and Dairy Queen and McDonald's opened.

The vitamins and minerals in plants were decreased due to farmers using fertilizers and irrigation to increase crop yields. Government support for soy and corn resulted in a a food industry with a huge monetary reason to use hydrogenated oils, high fructose corn syrup and modified corn starches to produce many highly processed, unhealthy foods. To offset these nutrient shortages the U.S. government issued guidelines to add vitamin B, iron riboflavin and thiamine to bread and other grain products.

These delights came into being in the 1940s.

M&Ms
Pillsbury cake mix
Cheetos

1950

A low point for American cuisine was this decade. Fast food restaurants sprouted up far and wide, and mass distribution of processed foods began with the advent of the new highways. The microwave was introduced for home use and did not add positively to America's health!

Pre-packaged foods were in high demand and busy housewives were elated to save time by using fast, canned and frozen foods. In 1958 the FDA's "Food Additives Amendment" required manufacturers to demonstrate the "safety" of new additives. (Yeah right!)

These delights came into being in the 1950s.

Swanson TV dinners
Cheez Whiz
Tang
Sweet 'n Low
Diet Rite

1960

The focus of the 1960s was on sweeping change and experimentation. Vegetarianism was catching on; fondue parties were popular and we returned to the outdoor cooking of our ancient forebears with the backyard barbecue. The first use of Aluminum cans for foods and beverages and irradiation of foods was done for the first time to stop sprouting, control insects and sterilize dried fruits and vegetables.

These delights came into being in the 1960s.

Tab and Diet Pepsi
Green Giant frozen veggies in butter sauce
Pringles
Gatorade

1970

In the 1970s economic problems meant homemade foods were simple. Consider Hamburger Helper and Betty Crocker's cookbook. Red Dye #2 was banned because studies indicated that it may cause cancer. As a result, red M&Ms disappeared for over a decade.

High fructose corn syrup became more and more predominant in drinks and processed foods. Products like "Miller Lite beer" were introduced to fight the extra weight average Americans were packing on.

These delights came into being in the 1970s.

Stove Top Stuffing
McDonald's Happy Meals
Hamburger Helper

1980

The 1980s were another depressing decade for "real food." The sadly missed red M&Ms returned. Aspartame an artificial sweetener was approved by the FDA. The USDA proclaimed that tomato sauce can be considered as a vegetable in school lunches. The first GMO crop, the tomato was developed and some new processed food stuffs were introduced to the market.

These delights came into being in the 1980s.

Lean Cuisine frozen dinners
Crystal Light powdered drink mix
Pop Secret Microwave Popcorn
Diet Coke

1990

Starting in 1990 the Nutrition Labeling and Education Act (NLEA) made it obligatory that all pre-packaged foods display standard nutrition labeling data.

The 1990s was also the decade that saw the first GMO foods in the market. Americans consumers purchased huge amounts of caloric sweeteners, and they were introduced to chips that contained Olestra.

2000

In the first decade of the second millennium the buzz words were "fat free", "low-fat" and "diet". Manufacturers lowered the fat content by taking out the high-fat ingredients, like oils and butters and preserved the flavor by adding preservatives, sweeteners, sugar and artificial flavors.

Gradually, food documentaries started to warn us of the hidden dangers in our foods and we began to ask how and where our food is produced. There was a veritable explosion of cooking programs on TV, inspiring us to prepare fresh foods at home. Organic foods went mainstream and large servings were on their way out. Super-fruits, like acai and pomegranate became household words and the FDA mandated that all food labels to include the content of trans-fats.

2010

And now, more than 100 years after processed foods were introduced and gained popularity, we once again find ourselves in an amazing age of real food, portion control, homegrown produce and food blogs.

THE PROBLEMS WITH PROCESSED FOODS

A few of the additives in processed foods are thought to compromise the structure of the body's and its function. It is suggested that they are related to the development of pulmonary, skin and psycho-behavioral disorders. Butylated hydroxytoluene (BHT) and butylated hydroxyanisole (BHA) are being studied for their possibility to damage genetic material thus promoting cancer. Sulfites are known to aggravate asthma in some youngsters and adults. Artificial colorings used in food, drinks and candy have been proven to cause allergic reactions in sensitive individuals stimulating conditions like ADHD, skin conditions and asthma. Hence, shunning foods containing these and various other chemical additives may significantly contribute to your health.

Artificial Sweeteners

The most commonly used artificial sweetener is the notorious compound called aspartame. Aspartame gains its notoriety because animal studies have proven that it can lead to the buildup of formaldehyde after ingestion, and one of the products produced as a result of aspartame in the intestine is a toxic compound called methanol. Low levels of aspartame have not pointed to direct symptoms so it is presumed safe in food products. However, this is a problematic because so many products contain aspartame. Hence, people who eat mainly processed foods are probably taking in rather high levels of aspartame. Little actual real data has been gathered to consider the level of aspartame consumed by an average person and how this level affects health, or the future effects in humans.

Artificial Coloring Agents

The majority of processed foods are colored with artificial coloring agents. The concept is that we eat with our eyes. Thus a lot of food producers choose to improve the color. Various kinds of coloring agents are used and these include many artificial compounds. Colorings are frequently often used to enhance the color of foods that lose color during storage or due to heat. The coloring agents in natural foods are very important phytonutrients and this loss of color often means a loss of nutritional value. This loss is covered up by the addition of artificial coloring compounds.

A large number of artificial colorings are a derivative of the manufacture of coal tars. Two of them are; FD&C Yellow#5, (tartrazine) and FD&C Blue#2 (indigo carmine). A few of these additives are known to promote allergic reactions in people, especially young children. In people who are sensitive, ingestion of these compounds has been linked to ADHD, asthma, and skin conditions such as urticaria and atopic dermatitis.

Preservatives

A huge worry with processed foods is preservative use. The most common preservatives are BHT and sulfites.

BHT = Butylated Hydroxytoluene

BHT is extremely provocative; a government-sponsored review of safety data in 1978 specified that no direct toxicity was perceived at the allowable levels in food. However, this report also noted that more studies were needed to evaluate safety. Following that study, BHT was been shown to promote stomach and liver tumors in when used in high amounts. The problem is that although this was permitted in foods at low levels for each food, it is present in many processed foods. Thus the amount consumed in one's normal diet may exceed the "safe" level and is still a concern for many scientists.

Both BHT and BHA (butylated hydroxyanisole) are being investigated due to their potential to damage genetic material. Also, current research is showing that they can rupture and damage one's red blood cells and stimulate symptoms of chemical sensitivity.

Sulfites

Sulfites are another common preservative. Sulfites are disallowed in foods that provide vitamin B1 because it can destroy this vitamin. Moreover, some people are sensitive to sulfites. People who are sensitive to sulfites respond with adverse reactions. Because of the reports of these adverse reactions, the use of sulfites on fruits and vegetables was banned by the FDA in

1986. The FDA is still reviewing whether or not sulfites should be banned from other uses also. Sulfites are known to exacerbate asthma in young children and adults. Somewhere between 5% and 10% of asthmatics are thought to be sulfite sensitive.

To learn more about sulfites visit

http://www.cfsan.fda.gov/~dms/fdpreser.html.

Pesticides

Organic foods are the safest and healthiest because they are not grown with chemical pesticides or fertilizers. The EPA (Environmental Protection Agency) believes a number of herbicides and fungicides to be possibly cancer causing. Most pesticides are known to cause some risk to humans. Some of those pesticides are organochlorines, organophosphates, organoarsenic and thiocarbamates.

On top of their potential to cause cancer, pesticides are believed to present distinct health threats to young so organic foods may be of supreme importance in protecting their health. The Environmental Working Group and the Natural Resources Defenses Council have established that millions of American children are subjected to levels of pesticides that go beyond limits believed to be safe. Some of these pesticides are neurotoxins. These neurotoxins can cause harm to developing brains and nervous systems. This is why they can be principally harmful to children. Also, researchers believe young children and adolescents may be particularly defenseless to the carcinogenic effects of some pesticides because our body is more sensitive to the effect of these chemicals during the time of growth and development.

Trans-Fats

Also known as hydrogenated fats, these fatty acids are in vegetable shortenings, margarine, cookies, crackers, snack foods and many other processed foods. The creation of trans-fats is accomplished by the chemical process of adding hydrogens to an unsaturated fatty acid. This process converts a liquid fat to a soft but solid form such as margarine. Trans-fats also increase the fats shelf-life.

Trans-fats elevate LDL cholesterol which is associated with the increased danger of heart disease and they decrease HDL cholesterol which is beneficial cholesterol. Trans-fats are also been linked to breast cancers.

A Practical Tip

All of these compounds are used just to make food look and taste as close to natural as possible. It is better to simply buy a natural, whole food and avoid these synthetics and get real food with the real benefits!

THE DANGERS OF PROCESSED JUNK FOODS

A leisurely walk down the aisles of your grocery store can be a pleasing experience. Many rows of appealing food wrapped up in vibrant packages, inviting you to try with snappy names and imaginative graphics.

Delicious food, that's pleasing to look at and convenient. Anything looking that lip-smacking has to be nutritious right?

Processed Foods Aren't only gotten from A Drive Thru.

The first picture that comes to most people's mind when they hear the phrase "processed food" is a burger and fries served at a fast food joint.

But the reality is that most of the food in your pantry is processed.

What Is Processed Food Anyway?

If it's canned, bagged, boxed or jarred and has a label with a list of ingredients, it's processed. The ways foods are processed include:

Canning
Freezing
Refrigeration
Dehydration
Aseptic Processing

All processed foods have been changed from their natural state for the reasons of "safety" and "convenience". And frightening as it appears, about 90% percent of the money spent on food goes on processed items.

Food Is Fine Just The Way It Is, Why Process It?

It all boils down to "convenience". It's much easier and faster to bake a cake by emptying a box, and adding an egg and some oil than it is to start from scratch.

Eating your noodles five minutes after pouring boiling water into the carton makes preparing lunch a breeze.

But you get far more than "convenience" by eating processed foods. There's slew of ingredients that manufacturers add. Here's a partial list:

Color to give your orange soda a nice glow
Stabilizers so your gravy isn't too watery
Emulsifiers to ensure the oil and water mix
Bleach it needs to be disinfected and deodorized

Texturizer - because nobody wants soggy cereal

Softeners - make it seem as though the ice cream was churned twice

Preservers - just in case you want to eat the cupcake in six months.

Sweetener - because sugar is sweet but saccharin and aspartame are sweeter.

Deodorizers - to remove the fish paste smell from your instant Pad Thai.

Flavor - to give you the sweet taste of fruit all year round.

Isn't that considerate of them!

If You Can't Say The Word, Do You Really Want To Eat It?

The big issue is that many processed foods have a list of ingredients similar to the list on a can of paint.

Look at this list of ingredients from strawberry flavoring for your milkshake:

Amyl acetate.
Amyl butyrate.
Amyl valerate.
Anethol.
Anisyl formate.
Benzyl acetate.
Benzyl isobutyrate.
Butyric acid.
Cinnamyl isobutyrate.
Cinnamylvalerate.
Cognac essential oil.
Diacetyl.
Dipropyl ketone.

Ethyl butyrate.
Ethyl cinnamate.
Ethyl heptanoate.
Ethyl lactate.
Etohyl methylphenylglycidate.
Ethyl Nitrate.
Ethyl propionate.
Ethyl valerbate.
Heliotropin.
Hydroxphrenyl-2butanone.
Isobutyl anthranilate.
Isobutyl butrate.
Lemon essential oil.
Maltol.
4-methylacetophenone.
Methyl anthranilate.
Methyl benzoate.
Methyl cinnamate.
Methyl heptine carbone.
Mthyl naphthyl ketone.
Methyl salicylate.
Mint essential oil.
Neroli essential oil.
Nerolin.
Neryl isobulyrate.
Orris butter.
Phenethyl alcohol.
Sore rum ether.
G-undecalctone.
Vanillin.
Solvent3.

Looks delightful, does it not? This is just a small sample of the 6,000 chemicals used to manufacture processed foods.

That Will Not Go In My Body!

Now you are probably thinking you have nothing to worry about, after all, you wouldn't even dream of drinking a milkshake or eating anything from a fast food restaurant. But it goes way beyond fast food.

What's In Your Pantry?

A study videotaped 32 families including dinner routines for 3 years. Even though 70% of these dinners were prepared at home, most included some packaged food. How many packaged foods do you use every day?

Always The Last To Know

There is no FDA requirement for food manufacturers to list the additives they use as ingredients that they consider "Generally Regarded As Safe" (GRAS). The label only has to say "artificial flavor" or "artificial coloring" or "natural" Yes, it can say "NATURAL".

Frozen Fish Sticks Have Never Killed Anybody

Here are a few things to consider before putting a jar of Vienna Sausages in your shopping bag:

Cancer - Some chemicals used in food processing are known to be carcinogenic.

A 7-year study conducted by the University of Hawaii which included 200,000 people established that the people who consumed the most processed meats had an almost 70% higher risk of pancreatic cancer than the people who ate none or very little processed meat products.

Obesity - Processed foods are normally higher in fat, sugar and salt. At the same time, they are lower in fiber and nutrients than the raw foods used to produce them. Thus processed foods are the ideal choice if you desire unhealthy weight gain and water retention.

The World Health Organization (WHO) has stated that processed foods are the cause of the spike rise of chronic disease and obesity levels around the world.

Heart Disease – Trans-Fatty Acids (TFA)are the dangerous type of fat you don't want to eat, yet many processed foods contain trans fatty acids. TFA's elevate the dangerous cholesterol, LDL, and quash the good one, HDL.

A recently conducted study at Harvard showed that the risk of heart disease was cut by 30% in women who avoided high-carb processed foods.

If That Won't Make You Avoid Processed Foods, Digest This:

Your taste buds become accustomed to the strong tastes of processed foods causing you to want to add more salt or sugar to the natural flavors of whole foods.

Some of these processed foods are full of unrecognizable parts and pieces, such as ears, snouts and esophagi!

To make up for the nutrients lost during processing, to "enhance" their nutritional content, synthetic vitamins and minerals are added.

If your diet is high in processed foods it can lead to diabetes, and liver overload.

OBESITY IS THE RESULT OF A DIET OF PROCESSED FOOD

According to a British BBC documentary aired in 2008 one in four preschool children in the UK were overweight or obese, these numbers closely matched childhood obesity in the United States.

The latest statistics show 30% of British children between 2 years and 15 years old are overweight or obese.

In the United States more than 33% of children and teenagers are either overweight or obese. Almost 20% of American children between 6 and 11 years old are categorized as obese. In 1980 that number was only 7%. Currently 5% of America's children are "severely obese," which puts them in the high risk group for chronic diseases normally found only in adults. Heart and liver disease are just two of them.

An interesting fact is that, unlike third-world countries, the poorest people in the United States are the most likely to be obese.

This apparent contradiction is a clear indication that the problem is with the diet. Some substance in the cheapest, most available foods is creating metabolic mayhem.

So it appears that this widespread obesity is the direct result of a diet of processed foods and their cheap artificial ingredients, non-nutritious fillers and synthetic chemical additives. Interestingly, many of these items are banned in other countries due to the negative health effects.

Virtually all processed foods are full of refined fructose, primarily in the form of high fructose corn syrup and in the United States, most of it is genetically engineered as an added bonus. This diet is a great recipe for obesity.

Obesity Is The Outcome Of A Processed Food Diet

Many parents are confused and befuddled about the reason for their child's excess weight. The cause of this problem becomes obvious when you start to take notice of the foods your child eats, and by the way, that includes baby food.

If you, like many mothers, feed your child baby food, infant formula, various fruit juices, you need to know that you are feeding your child massive amounts of sugar several times a day.

The reality is that some baby foods contain as much saturated fats and sugar as cheeseburgers and chocolate cookies. One survey conducted in 2009 that looked at over 100 foods for babies and toddlers found some were 29 percent sugar and others contained trans-fats which are linked to heart disease.

So it is inevitable that if a child starts out on a diet of processed fructose and trans-fats, that obesity will be the likely.

Parents need to wake up to the reality that there have been dramatic changes in processed foods over the years. The amount of processing and artificial chemical additives has greatly increased and most foods are now canned or boxed for your "convenience".

Today's packaged "convenience foods" have been processed and changed to the point of being effectively unrecognizable, nutrition wise, from the natural food.

Paul Gately, a Professor of Exercise and Obesity at Leeds Metropolitan University, says, it's vitally important to control your child's weight as early as possible, because obesity increases his/her risk of a wide variety of chronic diseases dramatically. These diseases include:

Diabetes, which leads to a host of other medical issues	Congestive heart disease, a disorder in which your heart can't pump enough blood
Pulmonary embolism, a likely fatal blockage	Fatty liver disease, when large pockets

of an artery	of fat build up in your liver cells
Osteoarthritis	Gout, a result of uric acid build up in your blood
Gallbladder disease, as a result of high cholesterol levels, which often causes gall stones	Cancer, particularly breast cancer

Are You Feeding Your Child Sugar All Day Long?

I totally disagree with the idea that young children are just eating too many calories and not getting enough exercise. Children have eaten with gusto for many centuries without suffering obesity and getting sick. The root of the problem lies in the source of the calories.

If you want your baby to have the best start nutrition wise, don't follow the advice given in a host of baby books telling you to feed your baby rice cereal which is a refined carbohydrate. Besides breast milk or formula, rice is the leading source of calories for infants in their first year and this is nothing short of a nutritional disaster.

For lots of children it's all downhill from there. Fructose, usually in some form of corn syrup, is now in almost every processed food and fast food you can imagine and fructose "programs" your body to consume calories and store fat.

Grains are other bad guys, because they are quickly transformed first into sugar and then into fat in your child's body. Fructose and grains affect the hormones insulin and leptin, both of which are very powerful fat regulators. So please don't be fooled into thinking that cereal is a good breakfast food. Kellogg, not so long ago had the impudence to claim that sugar does not cause Type II diabetes, obesity, hyperactivity or heart disease. They should have been fined for fraudulent advertising. Since then, they've recanted that crazy statement and now just want you to "put sugar in perspective," pointing out that:

"Sugar in cereals, including kids cereals, contributes less than 5 percent of daily sugar intake. Yet it adds taste, texture and enjoyment to cereal, while encouraging the consumption of fiber, vitamins and minerals; essential nutrients that you and your kids might not otherwise get from any other meal."

Kellog's contention is still absurd, because the nutrients your child requires are to be found in whole fresh foods; they will not be found in a box of processed cereal filled with sugar and synthetic chemical additives, but at least it's not blatantly deceitful like so many other food manufacturers who use outright lies and tricks to increase sales.

Many Kids Are Hooked On Soda And Sugary Fruit Drinks

Most children drink soda every day. A lot also drink "fruit juices," many of which contain only a small quantity, if any at all, actual fruit juice and tons of grams of sugar. Parents believe that fruit drinks are a healthy alternative for kids, and that is exactly what producers want them to believe. A recent report in the Guardian Express said; "kids are 40 percent heavier today compared to just 25 years ago, and a growing number of studies have linked rising childhood obesity rates to increased consumption of sugary beverages (including those sweetened with no- or low-cal sweeteners)".

The drink industry has denied its role in childhood obesity, in spite of the fact that they spend over $1 billion annually on youth-targeted marketing. The Guardian Express reported that 80% of American schools have agreements with either Coke or Pepsi to put their products in school vending machines. It's really an indefensible position. Obviously the marketing is effective or they wouldn't do it. When ads are targeted at an audience of 2 to 17-year-olds, it can hardly be considered an accident that kids in that age group choose soda whenever they're given a choice.

Children Are Also at Increased Risk from GMO Side Effects

Particularly in the United States, parents must contend with the fact that the majority of corn-based fructose is GMO and severely tainted with the toxic herbicide glyphosate. Glyphosate is the active ingredient in Monsanto's Roundup. Experts strongly believe that glyphosate is more toxic than the long banned product, DDT.

Persuasive evidence now indicates that glyphosate residues are found in most commonly eaten foods thanks to GMO sugar, soy, corn and wheat. These glyphosate residues augment the harmful effects of other food-borne chemical residues and toxins to disturb normal body functions and bring about disease. Glyphosate also upsets your gut flora, thereby further worsening metabolic mayhem and poor health.

Glyphosate, a pesticide containing carcinogenic properties seems to also be connected to autism. The active ingredient, Glyphosate is the primary chemical in Roundup. Round up is one of Monsanto's most indispensable products. Crops sold by the corporation are genetically-modified to resist the pesticide. A potential link has been identified between Glyphosate and cancer by The International Agency for analysis On Cancer.

Ingesting this poison, Glyphosate, however, could not be limited to cancer. According to analysis from one MIT scientist. 0.68% of children born in the U.S. have autism. It is believed that there is a link between autism and glyphosate. Dr. Stephanie Seneff, holds degrees in both biophysics and electrical engineering, however, of late her work has been concentrated on the link between nutrition and health.

Dr. Seneff strongly believes glyphosate could cause autism by disrupting gut bacteria. "The way glyphosate works is it interrupts the acid pathway, a metabolic function in plants that permits them to develop essential amino acids," Seneff explained at a recent Autism conference. Basically when this path is interrupted, the plants die. "Human cells don't have an acid pathway so scientists and researchers believed that exposure to glyphosate would be harmless. There is a problem with this theory. The problem is that bacteria have an acid pathway and we harbor millions of beneficial bacteria in our guts. They are known as our gut flora." These bacteria play a vital role in our health. Our gut is responsible for both digestion and our immune system. When glyphosate gets in our systems, it destroys our gut flora and our immune system. There is also a very strong probability that Glyphosate causes problems with vitamin D and liver function.

Glyphosate use in agriculture is linked to the increase of autism rates in the U.S. Jennifer Sass, in 2011, raised the alarm that glyphosate may be causing birth defects in humans.

As usual the U.S. government is doing nothing about this issue, so we have to take a stand and protect ourselves by not eating GM foods. Better yet, stop eating anything that comes from a factory.

Other GMOs (genetically modified organisms) are found in infant formulas, and nobody really knows yet what the long-term health risks of those ingredients might be. It's vital that we remember that infants experience greater exposure to chemicals than adults. Infants also have an immature and porous blood-brain barrier which allows more chemicals to reach their brains. Hence an all-organic diet is really crucial for infants and young children.

Breastfeeding: It Is the Healthy Start Your Baby Needs

Not only do many infant formulas lack the many of the critical nutrients obtained from breast milk, they also contain far too much sugar. Your baby does not need sugar. It's not only minerals, vitamins, proteins and fats that make mothers milk a healthier choice; breast milk contains substances that will considerably improve your child's gut and promote the healthy development of his/her nervous system.

If you are incapable of breastfeeding for any reason, you should consider purchasing human breast milk. Human breast milk is becoming a hot product online. Nursing mothers are now expressing and selling their extra milk to other families.

Whatever you do, try to avoid feeding your baby soy based formula. Soy based formula often contains extremely high concentrations of estrogenic compounds and manganese. It has also be found that infant formulas have been found to be tainted with a various of problematic chemicals. These chemicals include:

Perchlorates (used in rocket fuel).
Melamine.
Advanced glycoprotein end products.

How to Introduce Solid Foods

Putting breast milk aside, the food you prepare fresh as home are the best foods for your baby. The junk you buy in a store-cannot compare nutritionally, as they are often packed with unhealthy ingredients. When the time comes for your baby to start eating solids, present new foods one at a time 2 to 3 days apart. This way your baby gets accustomed to the food, and allows you to spot any food sensitivities and/or allergies. It is best to start with small serving sizes of just a spoonful or two.

As your infant develops you can evolve from pureed foods to finger foods he/she can feed him/her self. Just be sure the food is cut up small enough to not be a choking hazard. Nuts, popcorn, raisins and other small foods should be avoided due to the risk of choking.

Your Baby's Healthy Diet Is Up to You

Children will never know which foods are healthy foods if you as a parent don't teach them. Wholesome food is "live" and typically raw, and the guarantee of live food is that it will wilt and rot. Since burgers, buns, and fries do not decompose, even after a year, is an obvious indication that it's not real food and serves no nutritional purpose in your child's diet.

Kids need real nutrition, not the man-made chemicals that do not exists in natural food! These replacements are NOT equal to the real stuff.

Food is one component of the crucial lifestyle choices we first learn at home. Therefore it is important that you learn about proper nutrition and the dangers of junk food and processed foods. To provide your child with the best start in life, and help to introduce healthy habits that will last through their lives, you have to lead by example.

The easiest way back to good health for both children and adults alike, is to place your emphasis on whole foods that have not been changed from their original state or processed. Choose food that has been grown organically with no chemical additives, pesticides or fertilizers. Break free from the processed food diet that will inevitably make you sick.

Top 10 Cancer Causing Foods

The American Cancer Society now says your chances of getting cancer are 1 in 2 for men, and 1 in 3 for women!

Those shocking numbers point to a growing epidemic but it isn't time to cede the match. In an annual "cancer progress report", The American Association for Cancer Research said:

"it is estimated that more than 50 percent of the 585,720 cancer deaths expected to occur in the United States in 2014 will be related to preventable causes."

Since over 50% of cancers are avoidable, it seems that we need to take a closer look at we are subjecting out bodies to to see what might me a cause of this cancer epidemic. One of your obvious exposures to cancer is in what you eat. Cancer causing foods are probably in your diet every day and you don't realize it.

Here are 10 food products you should avoid.

Hydrogenated Oils

Hydrogenated oils and vegetable oils contain trans-fats. The Mayo Clinic says trans-fats are the worst type of fat there is. "Trans-fats are known to cause

heart disease, cancer and immune system problems",
said Dr. David Brownstein of News Mac Health. There
is no safe level of trans-fats in your diet. The FDA has
made an initial determination to say trans-fats are not
regarded as safe as they once thought. You should
avoid hydrogenated oil by choosing palm, coconut or
olive oil. Organic butter is also a better choice than
margarine.

French Fries/Potato Chips

French fries and potato chips are deep fried in
hydrogenated oil then heavily salted. The dangers of
hydrogenated oils is bad enough but the high salt
content is also very worrying. Excessive salt increases
the risk of high blood pressure and many other health
problems. Additionally, foods that have been heated
to high temperatures have high levels of acrylamide.
The National Cancer Institute stated that acrylamide
is found in both cigarette smoke and building
materials and in some foods. French fries and potato
chips have higher levels of this chemical that increases
the risk of cancer. Potatoes also have some of the most
pesticide residue of all the fruits and vegetables.

Microwave Popcorn

Most microwave popcorn contains more than just
kernels. It also contains perfluorooctanoic acid (PFOA)
which is a suspected carcinogen. Dr. Andrew Weil told
the world about microwave popcorn, saying artificial
butter contains a dangerous chemical that damages
your lungs when inhaled. To lower your risk of contact

with these chemicals, air pop your popcorn then add your own flavoring.

Processed Meats

Lunch meats, bacon, sausages, hot dogs and many other processed meats have been proven to give you a 67% increased risk of pancreatic cancer. More shocking information reveal hot dogs usually contain sodium nitrite. Sodium nitrite is a cancer causing chemical that the USDA has been trying to remove from the market since 70s. The risk of leukemia risks is a whopping 700% higher with hot dog consumption.

Red Meat

A new study has confirmed that red meat escalates cancer risks. The San Diego Union Tribune presented an article detailing study that showed that a sugar molecule, called Neu5Gc, joins with your body's own cells when red meat is eaten. Then your body attacks it, resulting in irritation and an increased risk of cancer. Previous studies have also shown an increase in breast cancer. You don't need to cease eating red meat completely. In fact, CNCA Health says "just opt for grass fed organic beef, which contains conjugated linoleic acids that actually fight against certain cancers". Also, keep red meat consumption to a minimum to further lower your risk.

Farmed Salmon

Some people, when avoiding processed and red meat, find themselves eating more salmon. Salmon is good but avoid the farmed version because a study at the University at Albany found it contains a lot cancer causing chemicals such as antibiotics, pesticides, PCBs, and flame retardants. To get the benefits of Omega 3 fatty acids that salmon gives you choose the wild Salmon without contaminants.

Refined Sugar/Soda

Refined sugar is dangerous because not only is it normally GMO but because it rapidly spikes blood glucose levels and this, in turn, feeds cancer cells. The type of sugar found in soda is Fructose. Fructose is a serious culprit for cancer too. Fructose contains caramel coloring which is a documented carcinogen. Soda also acidifies your body and acidification in turn causes cancer cells to multiply. Give sodas a total miss and limit your consumption of refined sugars.

Diet Foods

Whenever see the buzz words, "diet", "low-fat", "fat-free", or 'sugar-free" you can be sure those missing items have been replaced with chemical substitutes. Diet foods are packed with artificial sweeteners, colors and flavors. Saccharin, as the National Cancer Institute pointed out, was found to cause cancer in lab rats. Then there are the food dyes, "The three most widely used dyes, Red 40, Yellow 5, and Yellow 6, are contaminated with known carcinogens, says CSPI. Another dye, Red 3, has been acknowledged for years by the Food and Drug Administration to be a carcinogen, yet is still in the food supply." Choosing regular versions of these "diet" foods occasionally is better than the diet equivalents.

Refined White Flour

Bleaching food doesn't sound like a good idea because it isn't. Traces of the chemicals used to bleach the food remain in the food. Additionally, highly processed flours are high in carbohydrate content which upsets the blood sugar balance in our bodies leading to a higher output of insulin which in turn feeds cancer cells. Avoid highly processed carbohydrates such as white pasta, white bread, soda, white rice and concentrated fruit juices.

GMOs/Glyphosate

Since the FDA does no testing to ensure safety, GMOs have made their way into most of our foods. GMO foods have been altered to tolerate heavy doses of glyphosate, the chemical found in Round-Up, OR have been re-engineered to hold a toxin that kills pests. Insufficient independent (non-Monsanto) studies have been done to truly determine the safety or the danger, but so far independent testing has shown GMO's to cause speedy tumor growth in lab rats. At this time, GMOs are not required to be disclosed on food labels in the US. Glyphosate, which is the most often used pesticide sprayed on crops has been linked to intestinal discomfort, Non-Hodgkin's Lymphoma and birth defects among other things.

Choosing only certified organic food is the only way to avoid GMOs and pesticides.

Do Processed Foods Raise The Risk Of Autoimmune Disease?

If you are struggling to eat healthier, a study published in the journal Autoimmunity Reviews may help you get back on track. Researchers have suggested that eating processed foods can weaken your intestines in a manner that increases your risk of autoimmune diseases like celiac disease, Type I diabetes and multiple sclerosis.

Researchers have already identified at least 7 food additives that have been shown to weaken the intestine's immune response to toxins. This condition it is thought, could lead to autoimmune diseases.

Following a long, hard day at work, it is appealing to choose foods that are quick and easy to prepare. This, for many people, means they choose processed foods like microwave meals. Microwave meals are typically high in salt, fat, sugar and other less than desirable additives.

Many studies have documented the negatives of eating some processed foods. These negatives include an increased risk of weight gain and heart disease. Recently WHO (World Health Organization) determined that colorectal cancer can be caused by eating processed meats.

Now, Dr. Torsten Matthias, of the Aesku-Kipp Institute in Germany and Prof. Aaron Lerner, of the Technion-Israel Institute of Technology in Haifa, Israel have suggested that eating many of these "processed" foods might be associated with development of autoimmune diseases.

At least seven identified food additives appear to weaken the intestine's ability to resist toxins

Autoimmune diseases occur when your immune system attacks healthy cells because they mistake them for foreign invaders. This often leads to the destruction of body tissue along with anomalous organ growth and function.

Some Fast facts about processed foods

Currently over 75% of the sodium consumed by Americans consume derives from processed and restaurant foods

Any food that displays a nutrition label can generally be considered as being processed

Not all food processing is bad. For example, milk needs to be pasteurized to remove harmful bacteria.

Learn about healthy eating

There are in excess of 100 autoimmune disorders. The more common and well known ones include Type I diabetes, celiac disease, multiple sclerosis (MS), rheumatoid arthritis and Crohn's disease.

Professor Lerner and Doctor Matthias noted a connection in recent years between the rise of the incidence of autoimmune diseases and the consumption of processed foods. For their study, they decided to determine whether or not there is a link between the two.

Specifically, they looked at how certain additives used to improve the texture, taste, smell and shelf life, affect the intestines and the progress of autoimmune diseases.

In their study, they found at least 7 food additives, including gluten, glucose, fat solvents, sodium, nanometric particles, organic acids and microbial transglutaminase that weakened tight junctions in the intestine.

Based on these findings, they suggested that the consumption of processed foods probably increases the risk of autoimmune diseases. They noted that the food additive market is under regulated, making such discoveries a cause for concern.

Professor Lerner says: "Control and enforcement agencies such as the FDA stringently supervise the pharmaceutical industry, but the food additive market remains unsupervised enough. We hope this study and similar studies increase awareness about the dangers inherent in industrial food additives, and raise awareness about the need for control over them."

The FDA, in June of 2015, revealed they are going to ban a significant source of artificial trans-fats called partially hydrogenated oils (PHOs), with the hope that doing so will reduce the risk of heart attacks and heart disease for Americans.

How Processed Foods Affect Your Health

Processed foods = foods that have been altered by adding hormones, additives, unnatural genetic material, preservatives or various other chemical or heat treatments that change or destroy fatty acids, natural healthy enzymes, vitamins and minerals.

The driving motivator of food processing is extending the shelf life of foods.

In dissimilarity, whole foods are unpretentious and basic. Whole foods do not require processing. Whole foods can be eaten off the vine or off the fire. Like you and I, whole foods age so they must be eaten when fresh.

A List of Processed Food

Did you ever notice that the ingredients in processed foods are cloaked in mystery? Food manufacturers patent some of their processing methods. As an example, the procedure for making Splenda is a big secret patented with the US Government.

I would think that if you need to keep secret how a food is made, it probably indicates that if most people knew how it was done, they wouldn't eat it.

This is a very short list of some common processed foods:

White wheat flour, especially bleached.
Refined sugars.
Margarine and other hydrogenated vegetable fats.
Refined vegetable oils.
Artificial sweeteners.
Food additives.
Canned foods.
Boxed foods such as meal mixes, cereal and pasta.
Soft drinks and sugary "fruit" drinks.
Fast food, a source of trans fats.
Cheese food.
Packaged cakes and cookies.
Chips.
Snack food crackers and other junk food
Processed meat products if they contain artificial colors and soy fillers.
Frozen foods like tv dinner meals.
Fish sticks.
Pizza rolls and similar foods
Soy products.
Powdered milk and eggs.

Processed food has been modified extensively from its natural state.

Other Less Obvious
Processed Foods to Avoid

Stay away from non-organic pasteurized, homogenized milk and any products derived from it.

Many dairy farms inject their milking cows with rBGH (recombinant bovine growth hormone) which is created from GMOs. rBGH increases the milk production but also afflicts the cows, increasing by 40-55%, both udder infections and lameness.

Interestingly, rBGH has been banned in Canada, Europe, Japan, Australia every other industrialized nation but not in the United States. (What's up with that?)

In pasteurized milk, the proteins have been changed by the high heat applied and likewise the good digestive enzymes and vitamins have been ruined. Without the good enzymes, milk is much harder to digest and the result is "lactose intolerance".

You should never buy meat, poultry or pork from "factory farms". Here's the reason: The animals raised in these environments are abused, confined, fed food which makes them sick (GM soybeans and corn, bakery waste, other dead animals, manure and other sickening things). Many become very ill from this ill-treatment.

They are injected with anti-bacterial drugs, further contaminating their flesh. What's worse is that this reliance on drugs is an invitation to the growth of new and lethal bacteria strains that are impervious to modern antibiotics. It is better to choose grass fed, organic meats and true free range chicken instead.

Processed foods are made not to benefit you, rather they are made for convenience and long shelf life. Real nutrition draws the short straw in the methods used to create these foods. Thus the relationship between processed food and good health is not a favorable one.

If the loss of nutrition during production wasn't bad enough, most of the convenience foods suggest using a microwave oven to heat them, the microwave simply further depreciates any nutritional value.

Food Additives

Processed foods have huge amounts of food additives. Some of these additives are relatively harmless, but many have unwelcome health effects.

Food additives are materials that manufacturers add to a widespread range of foods to either preserve the flavor or improve the taste and visual appeal of the foods. They are very common in foods which need long shelf lives and they are used extensively in "diet" foods, which require a flavor boost.

A few additives are derived from natural sources, but most are highly processed substances developed from less than healthy sources such as coal tar and peroxide.

Genetically Engineered Foods

If you need a sobering factoid; nearly 75% of the processed foods found in your local grocery store contain soybean, corn or canola ingredients that have been engineered from GMOs. The list includes corn products, baked goods, salad dressings, infant formula, baby food and various other products.

Common vegetables like tomatoes and potatoes are also being treated to GMO. Just recently, the bio-tech companies have requested permission to genetically alter fish. As hard as it may be to believe, a company in Japan is already marketing fruit flavored fresh fish. They are transforming that flavor by feeding the farmed fish food containing artificial flavors. Gives new meaning to Orange Roughy huh?

Farmers have reported that livestock will ignore genetically engineered corn in favor or naturally raised corn when given a choice. That should convey a message.

Now, the bulk of this information is not "scientific" but common sense dictates that if cows won't ingest genetically engineered food crops by choice, and insects die after intermingling with them, it would seem to be wise to avoid them whenever you can.

Our bodies did not evolve eating these hi-tech foods, and the negative health results have been well documented in many studies.

Keep in mind that by shunning processed junk foods, you will avoid most genetically engineered foods.

A Few Thoughts

It is not my intent to convey that junk food is evil or is to be avoided at all costs.

Some food processing is beneficial because it helps to neutralize any natural toxins in food before they are consumed.

There are times that you just want to eat something because you enjoy the taste. Eating a small amount of processed occasionally won't have a great effect on your overall health.

But, a incessant diet of junk food will have an effect on your well-being and long-term risk of disease.

Foods such as open range, grass fed meats, poultry, eggs, fresh organic vegetables and fruit, tropical oils, wild caught seafood, clean, raw diary products and properly prepared nuts and grains will support the growth and preservation of your muscles and organs.

Make these types of foods the bulk of your meals, and you'll accomplish a lot in avoiding the health problems connected to non-nutritious, processed junk foods.

WHAT PROCESSED FOODS ARE DOING TO KIDS

Being a parent, I find avoiding processed food to be a real trial. Going to the health food stores to fill my pantry doesn't solve the problem. I want my kids to eat natural, healthy food, but processed look alluring, especially with young children. They're generally quite cheap, not always, but often. And then there's the advertising aspect. If I give my children a choice between a box of crackers that look like fish and an apple, they'll choose the cute little fish no matter how much I go on about the benefits of kiwi.

The solution really is very simple. When the kids are young: either don't give them a choice or just refuse to buy it when they ask. But you say, "what about when they get older and are out there on their own?" Some people might believe it is silly to be anxious about eating processed food with all the other pressures of life, but a diet of mainly processed food has substantial effects on one's health during childhood, adolescence, and teenage years. Here's a few of the health concerns processed food has been connected to in children:

ADHD: In 2011 a randomized organized trial circulated in the Lancet, "children with ADHD who eliminated processed food showed a significant decrease in ADHD symptoms. When the foods were reintroduced, symptoms intensified."

Type II Diabetes: A study published in the proceedings of the National Academy of Sciences stated, "processed foods contribute to the development of insulin resistance due to their concentrations of chemicals called advanced glycation endproducts, or AGEs."

Autism: In 2012 a study distributed in Clinical Epigenetics discovered that excessive consumption of additives like high fructose corn syrup, leads to mineral deficits that might lead to autism.

Obviously these studies have limitations but it certainly appears to be the case that raising kids on a highly processed diet has consequences for their future health. But there's a fundamental question here; what exactly is processed foods? Gogurt and Snackables are obvious examples, but it gets vague when you consider that the majority of foods found in a grocery store that are packaged.

Here is a list of what I consider the top ten offenders when you are determining how processed a food is. The next time your child begs for a fancy packaged delight, take a look at the food label and see if it contains any of the following:

High fructose corn syrup
Trans fat
Partially hydrogenated oil
Monosodium glutamate (MSG)
Textured protein
Hydrolyzed protein

Artificial colors
Brominated vegetable oil
Artifical sweeteners/sugar alcohols
Various offensive oils (corn oil, palm oil, soybean oil)
Wheat flour
Nitrates/nitrites
Butylhydroxytoluene, or BHT

This list is just the beginning, there are sadly many more long lists we could create. But besides nutrition labels, I have learned that avoiding processed food isn't just about rejecting ingredients. If you really want to not feed your children processed food, you have to change the way you look at food and its preparation. Moving away from processed food in our family, has only been one small part of a complete process of appreciating food together as a family. It's about attentive eating and sensible food choices.

The next time you think about grabbing a sugary snack for your child, ask yourself "why am I making this choice?" If it's because you're short of time or you're looking for something you can use as a bribe, take a minute to consider that stimulus. You, as a parent, are responsible for your child's health and well-being.

SALT IS STILL HIGH IN FAST AND PROCESSED FOODS

Fast-food restaurants provide filling, cheap meals and quick snacks. But there is always a hidden additional cost: a dollop of salt that isn't good for heart health. Regardless of the current outcry for reducing salt in the American diet, and manufacturers vowing to do just that, the amount of salt in processed foods hasn't changed very much since 2005.

So, you ask, why does salt matter? Too much salt in your diet can increase blood pressure and force your kidneys to work harder. High blood pressure is a leading cause of heart attack, stroke, kidney disease, heart failure and more. The most current recommendations advise us to consume no more than 2,300 milligrams of salt per day. That is equal to about a teaspoon of table salt. The recommendation is lower for people with cardiovascular disease or high blood pressure, then it is no more than, 500 mg a day. However, the average American is consuming, on average, 3,400 mg a day.

Researchers at Harvard recently made a study that calculated the cumulative health effects of excessive salt intake. They determined that excessive salt intake is responsible for 2.3 million deaths each year. The U.S. placed 19th of the 30 biggest countries, with 429 deaths per million. That signifies 1 out of 10 U.S.

deaths due to stroke, heart attack and other cardiovascular diseases.

Counting the milligrams

For the JAMA Internal Medicine study, researchers with the Center for Science in the Public Interest (CSPI) in Washington, DC, assessed the salt in 78 foods served at fast food restaurants between 2005 and 2011 by gathering nutritional data from the company websites. They did the exact same thing for foods picked from shelves at stores in Washington, DC, and at a Walmart in Elverston, Pennsylvania.

The average salt content in chain restaurants increased by 2.6% from 2005 to 2011 while in packaged foods, it fell an average of 3.5%. The salt in some foods fell as much as 30%, however, a greater number went up by more than 30%.

CSPI, which backed the study, has called for tighter regulation on the salt content in processed and fast food restaurants. They suggest phasing in ever-stricter limits on what quantity of salt foods may contain.

Michael F. Jacobson, Ph.D., and colleagues, wrote "Stronger action...is needed to lower sodium levels and reduce the prevalence of hypertension and cardiovascular diseases."

When it is applied to millions of people, even slight changes in salt consumption saves lives. Dr. Dariush Mozaffarian, associate professor of medicine at Harvard-affiliated Brigham and Women's Hospital says "The evidence is convincing that substantially reducing sodium intakes from current levels will have significant population benefits."

How to reduce your Salt

There is no need to wait for more regulations to reduce the sodium in your diet. Dr. Helen Delichatsios, an assistant professor of medicine at Harvard Medical School says "Eat out less and cook at home more. There is much less sodium in home cooking than in prepared or restaurant foods."

When shopping, always check the nutrition labels and use less foods that deliver a lot of salt. The top 5 processed food sources of salt are cold cuts and cured meats, bread and rolls, poultry, pizza and soups. The best however is simply avoid labeled foods and eat real food like vegetables, fruits, whole grains and legumes says Dr. Delichatsios.

If you are dining out, ask for information on fat, calories and salt. Commonly, chain restaurants post the nutrition of their products online.

Cook more. Plan your meals based on fresh, whole foods that you cook at home rather than processed heat-and-serve products because they have a tendency to be loaded with salt.

Top 10 Food And beverage Manufacturers

The list includes all of the big names. While consumers might not recognize names like JBS USA or ConAgra, they do know the consumer brands these companies produce. JBS USA produces Swift meats and ConAgra produces Healthy Choice and Chef Boyardee - to name just a few.

General Mills, Inc.

General Mills markets many well-known brands, including Betty Crocker, Yoplait, Colombo, Totino's, Pillsbury, Green Giant, Old El Paso, Häagen-Dazs, Cheerios, Trix, Cocoa Puffs, and Lucky Charms. General Mills portfolio includes more than 90 other leading brands

Kraft Foods, Inc.

Kraft Foods core businesses are in cheese, dairy foods, beverage, snack foods and fast foods. Some of Kraft's major brands are;

Vegemite, A.1., Grey Poupon, Gevalia, Planters, Capri Sun, Jell-O, Kraft, including Kraft Dinner, Kraft Singles, Kraft Mayo, Maxwell House, Oscar Mayer, Polly-O, Velveeta, RIDG's Finer Foods, licensing name used by Kraft addressing Bull's-Eye Barbecue Sauce, Kool-Aid and Boca Burger.

In 2013, Vani Hari and Lisa Leake began an online drive to force Kraft Foods Group to remove synthetic dyes from its macaroni and cheese products.

In April 2013, Hari and Leake delivered a petition with over 270,000 signatures to Kraft in Chicago, requesting the company to change its macaroni and cheese recipes.

In October 2013, Kraft promised to remove artificial dyes from three macaroni and cheese products in kid-friendly shapes, but not from its elbow-shaped Kraft Macaroni and Cheese product.

ConAgra Foods, Inc:

ConAgra produces many food products including cooking oil, frozen dinners, hot cocoa, hot dogs, peanut butter and a host of others. The major brands under ConAgra's banner are: Healthy Choice, Hunt's, Healthy Choice, Orville Redenbacher, Marie Callender's, Reddi-wip, Slim Jim (snack food), Egg Beaters, P.F. Chang's Home Menu, Hebrew National and Bertolli ready meals.

Anheuser-Busch InBev

Anheuser-Busch InBev is the largest beer company with over 200 beer brands brewed and marketed throughout the world. A-B Inbev's global brands are Corona, Budweiser, Beck's, Stella Artois, Leffe and Hoegaarden. The other brands which are too many to list, are categorized as local brands.

Coca Cola, Co.

Coca Cola brands are too multitudinous to list if you want to know what they are visit this page: https://en.wikipedia.org/wiki/List_of_Coca-Cola_brands

JBS USA.

A leading processor of pork, beef and lamb in the U.S. and Canada

NESTLE

Like Coca Cola, Nestle's list is too long to include. You can view it here: http://www.nestle.com/brands/brandssearchlist

TYSON FOODS, INC.

Tyson Foods is the world's second largest processor and marketer of chicken, beef, and pork after JBS S.A. Tyson Foods exports the largest percentage of beef out of the United States. It operates major food brands, including Hillshire Farm, Jimmy Dean, Sara Lee, Ball Park, Wright, State Fair and Aidells.

PEPSICO, INC.

PepsiCo's products include: Pepsi, Diet Pepsi, Mountain Dew, Lay's, Gatorade, Tropicana, 7 Up, Doritos, Lipton Teas, Brisk, Quaker Foods, Cheetos, Mirinda, Ruffles, Aquafina, Naked, Kevita, Propel, Sobe, H2oh, Sabra, Starbucks (ready to Drink Beverages), Pepsi Max, Tostitos, Mist Twist, Fritos, and Walkers.

A Preview Of:
Common Sense Life Hacks

*A Survival Guide to Achieving Your Goals
And Improving Your Business And
Personal Relationships*

A.L.Harlow

INTRODUCTION

Everybody wants to succeed in life. Success is everybody's dream. Unfortunately though, it is not presented on a silver platter. The pursuit of success is the driving factor of most people's lives. Humans simply want better in their lives.

This book contains two hundred tips to help you to better your life and improve personal and business relationships. If you follow these tips you will be empowered and equipped to attain whatever realistic goals you set.

Here's some simple advice that has been given to many people; "If you do as you've always done you will get as you've always gotten."

The Grand Idea

Maintain The Proper Mindset

The right attitude must be maintained whether you are building a business or driving to work. Maintaining a good attitude is and always will be the number one precondition for achieving your goals. And frankly, it is the sole qualification that you will need.

Be Interested And Listen

Knowledge is power and if you are not listening, you will lack knowledge. Without knowledge you quite simply will have no direction. You don't have to know everything but it matters a lot to know what does matter.

Maintain Your Good Health

Do not be silly enough to think that you can make it on intelligence alone. Consume proper amounts of food and water. If you neglect your health you can never accomplish your goal.

Use Your Common Sense

Here's a truth that smarts to hear or read about. Data has piled up on the amount of people who lose everything they have because they didn't use common sense. It is pre-programmed into everybody and using it actually makes life in general much easier.

Smile a Lot

It's true! Smiling goes above almost all differences. Just think how much it would benefit your cause. It is not the most trivial of signals. Smiling is something that works to your benefit. This has been proven time after time.

For more books by this author, please go to:
www.Al-Harlow.com